Intermittent Fasting For Women: The No-Bullshit Guide To Effortless Fat Loss

Joe Petrakovich

May 3, 2016

Contents

0.1 Copyright

0.2 Medical Disclaimer

Although the author and publisher have made every effort to ensure that the information in this book was correct at press time, the author and publisher do not assume and hereby disclaim any liability to any party for any loss, damage, or injury caused by errors or omissions, whether such errors or omissions result from negligence, accident, or any other cause.

This book is not intended as a substitute for the medical advice of physicians. The reader should regularly consult a physician in matters relating to his/her health and particularly with respect to any symptoms that may require diagnosis or medical attention.

Part I

The Reasoning

Chapter 1

Why Does This Book Exist?

Welcome!

Greetings and congratulations for taking action towards the benefit of your health. Perhaps you bought this book because you've heard about this thing called intermittent fasting and how awesome it can be, but found that all the information seems to be written for male gym bros and beef-cake body builders.

Maybe you've gotten the impression that only men get to experience this "effortless" weight loss, and that women drew the short end of the stick because of genetics related to pregnancy.

Or perhaps you were like me 5 years ago and you already know the basics of intermittent fasting, but you're not sure how you can fit it into your life TODAY.

There could be countless reasons why you decided to read this book but, nonetheless, you've made a great decision. When you finish reading, you'll be able to integrate intermittent fasting into your daily life and reap the benefits immediately. You'll be able to tell your friends about it in a simple, non-scientific way that JUST MAKES SENSE. You won't have any doubt that women too can experience a much easier way to lose weight without having to eat only salads (I mean unless you want to...).

And, no, the bread and butter of intermittent fasting is not about weird scientific "tricks". Here we are going to cut to the chase and deliver you real, practical, essential strategies to help you finally get the body you want.

Chapter 2

My Background And Why You Should Practice Intermittent Fasting

So, I'd like to offer you a little bit of my background so you can get a feel for why intermittent fasting has been so valuable to me.

I grew up in the kind of household where dinner time was one of the only occasions when my brother and I could please our father. We did this by being animated about how good the food was, and having seconds, thirds, and even four plates of food. I got accustomed to thinking that being really full meant that you had eaten enough.

I've been overweight my whole life until now. My relationship with food just wasn't good. I was a classic emotional eater.

Eventually, I got serious about my weight and, investigator that I am, researched all the best diets and tricks in the book. I tried being vegan, pescetarian, strange lemonade "cleanses", mindful eating, and paleo. The best I could seem to do was hover around 200 lbs. (still uncomfortably chubby) while eating paleo. What kept resurfacing was my relationship with food, and the weekly binge would continuously throw me off track. All the above methods actually worked for a little while, but it was my own mind that kept sabotaging my efforts.

About 5 years ago, I got serious. I hired a diet coach who had me doing everything from heavy weight training to macro-nutrient cycling, and intermittent fasting. This is where I first learned about intermittent fasting. I approached my ideal weight with him, but I inevitably gained some of weight back because I hadn't dealt with a core problem. What I did notice, though, was that my weight seemed to finally level off and never rose back to those ungodly levels prior to that.

What kept it down? Intermittent fasting! This was simply due to that classic equation, my eating window being later in the day; I just couldn't put down enough food to gain weight. I would still have an occasional screw up, but my weight wouldn't spiral out of control.

Now, this isn't an excuse to eat poorly, but rather to signify the first realization of the usefulness of intermittent fasting.

2.1 Eating... Continued

I ate this way for about 5 years, with spurts of enthusiasm here and there on really reaching my goal weight, but it wasn't enough. I was still eating quite a bit of food, more than I needed. Intermittent fasting, and about 80% low-carb paleo helped to keep my weight from surging, but that's about it.

Finally, we get to today. I noticed, while on a trip to Texas, my weight started going up unusually. I gained 5 then 10 pounds over a few weeks. I wasn't sure what was going on, but I knew I had slacked on my diet. I was eating more fast food than usual and not moving very much at all.

Fortunately for me, this weight surge was the kick in the ass I needed to finally get serious. I needed a solid plan, based on tested fat loss techniques, and I needed to stick to it. Luckily, intermittent fasting had grown in popularity over the 5 years and I was able to find a simple solution, the one I will present in this very book. It's a way to eat less food so that fat is lost, but be able to eat large satisfying meals. A solution based on simplicity, presented clearly, and without excessive measurement and tracking.

Chapter 3

A Brief Introduction To Intermittent Fasting

You may have heard about intermittent fasting from your friends, or maybe some random talk show mentioned it as some fat loss miracle. You've overheard some bros at the gym bringing it up during their chat about carb-cycling and protein shakes. But what is it really?

The name says it all. Intermittent - periods of time; fasting - being without food. What's so special about periods of time without food? Every time I say the word fasting to my relatives, they get this big fearful look on their face as if I am starving myself and could die at any moment!

Fortunately, you won't be starving yourself. It's not one of those fasts that last 30 days and have you drinking lemonade and spices.

In essence, intermittent fasting is a strategy to make dieting easier. How does it do that? Well, let's define dieting. I'll bring this up again later, but, in order to lose weight, you simply have to eat less than you are eating right now. That's a challenge for people because the usual method people take is to start giving up the things that they love. They start eating tiny salads, give up their cheeseburgers, and it starts to become painful. So what happens? They fail. We have all done it. You want to be healthy, but your day is already full of stress, and food is your outlet (well, it's mine anyway!), it helps you wind down.

This is where the magic of intermittent fasting can save the day. Don't eat after dinner until the following day at lunch, shifting your eating into a smaller window of time.

What does this do? It lets you eat big, satisfying meals, but is ultimately less food than you would normally eat. And boom! Dieting is not so hard after all.

Now, I know, I'm leaving out lots of details. You might be shouting at this book right now thinking, *No, breakfast is IMPORTANT! Fasting will put my body in starvation mode!* Don't worry; we will clear up that nonsense in the coming chapters.

Chapter 4

The Real, Tangible, Everyday Benefits

4.1 It Isn't A Trick, It Just Makes Dieting Easier

Despite all of the scientific jargon you may have heard about intermittent fasting (or IF as I will now refer to it from here on out), the actual benefits you inherit are far simpler and more practical. Yes, some studies show that mice live longer, but what does that mean for you and your goals?

By and far, the most real and immediate benefits from IF are that it makes dieting EASIER. I'll explain why:

You and I both know that to lose weight, you have to eat less or move more, or both at the same time. This has been the case since the beginning of time. Virtually all diets achieve this in some way. The paleo diet, for example: eliminate all processed food and grains. When it comes down to it, most weight lost on this diet is simply because you are eating less (you have practically eliminated an entire food group).

How does intermittent fasting help you eat less? Well, you are eliminating breakfast! By refraining from food until lunch, you have a smaller window of time to eat for the day, making it much easier to eat less than normal and thereby lose weight!

Now, I know what you are thinking:

But...breakfast is the most important meal of the day!

This is a statement that has probably been ingrained into your head your entire life but, as nutrition science has grown over the years, this one has become relegated to the book of myths. The only studies that show breakfast as beneficial are correlative, not causative, which basically means that it was shown that healthy people tend to eat breakfast, so perhaps breakfast is what makes them healthy. The real truth to this study is simply that people who eat breakfast have stabler, less stressful, scheduled lives, so they are healthier because of their ability to manage themselves. It's also a statement that has grown so large because of the marketing efforts of cereal companies, rather than its usefulness to you and me.

Okay, so you're going to start skipping breakfast, and you're probably wondering, *Won't I be starving? How will I go about my day without being a hot mess at work?*

Okay, here's the deal: the reason you wake up hungry is mostly due to a hormone response. Now, it's possible you don't wake up hungry, since many people aren't hungry in the morning naturally. If that's not you, then you probably tend to eat breakfast around the same time every morning, so your body sends a signal every morning to keep this pattern going. In order to start practicing intermittent fasting, you'll have to adjust. That means about 1 to 2 weeks where you'll feel hungry and you'll have to push through it. Don't worry; it's not that bad, and later in this book I'll offer some strategies that make it a breeze. You'll wonder why you haven't been doing this your whole life.

Once you've grown accustomed to breakfast skipping, and pushing your usual eating to later in the day, making it easier to eat LESS, you'll be well on your way to reaching your weight loss goals. All that's left is consistency. In subsequent chapters I'll discuss a typical diet setup and what you can expect over time. Fortunately though, the benefits are not only about weight. The reason intermittent fasting has been such a hit these past couple years is because the benefits go beyond the scale and into the realm of psychology, productivity, and even saving you a few bucks.

4.2 Psychological Benefits: The Mental Game Of Dieting

If you're like me, you love food. I mean LOVE it. Who wants to eat salads every day? Not me. Hey, there's nothing wrong with a good salad but, in my opinion, if you are going to be consistent with your diet – and you will need to be in order to be successful - you have to be able to enjoy what you are doing. If you have to eat tiny salads and chicken breast every day, you're going to struggle. You'll be stressed out; you'll get bored; you'll screw up. Here's how IF helps: because you have shifted your eating window to later in the day, you get to eat BIG, satisfying meals. It's quite difficult to overeat 1800+ calories in an 8-10 hour window unless you really try or are eating garbage in the first place. On that note, it's important to remember that this isn't an excuse to eat junk. Junk still adds up quickly. But it does give you a lot of leeway to eat the meals you like, and to eat until you are full. This is one of the main benefits people rave about with IF; you are on a diet but it doesn't look or feel like it because you get to eat big. Screw the salads; go for the steak and potatoes.

Another benefit is helping to remove obsessiveness about food and what to eat. People practicing IF report that fasting has helped refresh their outlook on food as more of a fuel source rather than a stress relief. You'll learn your body's true signals for hunger and when you really need food, rather than just your conditioned response.

In the morning hours, while you're sipping your black coffee, you won't feel lethargic and slow for your usual bagel and cream cheese. Instead, you'll be focused and alert, being more effective, efficient, and productive.

Finally, and this has been one of my favorites, you'll have one less meal to shop for. This doesn't mean you never get to eat breakfast again. That would be ridiculous ... we both know breakfast food rocks. But cutting out breakfast has simplified my life immensely. I buy a third less groceries, plan a third less meals. Time saved. Money saved. What could be better than that?

Of course, if you have a family, and they don't all practice IF, well, you might be out of luck on some of those benefits, but maybe you can convert them!

Part II

The Plan

Chapter 5

What Works For Me And The Results You Can Expect

A common question I am asked is, "What kind of results will I see?" No one wants to make a change to their life without knowing the kind of success they could have and how fast it will come.

When it comes to weight loss, it's always a mixed bag. If you've been eating garbage your entire life, full of salt and sugar, you'll probably drop weight fast. If you are holding a lot of water, you can drop literally 10 pounds in less than a week.

But when we are talking about fat loss, it all depends on the classic calories in/calories out equation. Later we will go over a way to get a baseline diet in place. For now, I'll show you what I have done in the past and the typical results that I saw by outlining a day-in-the-life scenario.

5.1 Morning (7-9am)

I wake up and have a 16oz. black coffee and sip it with some water while I do my morning routine- usually clearing my email, balancing my budget, and tying up any loose ends from the previous day. Stuff I like to do. Fasting and drinking coffee powers me through the morning. I feel lightweight and on point, a notable difference compared to when I ate breakfast. Eating breakfast would leave me feeling sluggish and bloated.

5.2 Noon (12-1pm)

While my co-workers are shoving food in their faces, I take this time to go on a brisk walk. I'm still feeling sharp at this point, and fasted, steady-state cardio like walking will be fueled by body fat, exactly what I want. When the walk is over, I'm vibrating with energy and I feel great. The exercise also suppresses any hunger pangs I might have otherwise had.

5.3 Afternoon (1-3pm)

This is where *before using the style I outline in this book* I would eat my first big meal. Now, however, I have learned to stretch it a bit further. If I feel hungry or am noticing a performance decrease in my work, I'll have a small apple, or sip a seltzer water. The apple will give me plenty of energy to make it to 3 or 4pm to have my first meal. This is just how I do it, feel free to eat a little earlier or later. For me, eating the first meal as late as possible without getting grumpy or tired makes it so I'm no longer hungry until bed time (or later). This is the best way I can keep my calories low for fat loss.

5.4 Night: (6-11pm)

I'm usually nice and satisfied from my meal and don't think about food again for the rest of the day. I'll have my small meal near bed time when I feel some hunger, and that's it!

Following this plan, with the amount of food I like to eat, I end up taking in about 1800-1900 calories. For my weight, this results in about 1-2 pounds of fat lost per week. When I hit the weight I like, I increase my food intake so that I maintain the weight. This usually means eating a slightly larger second meal, perhaps doubling it in size.

Simple and straightforward. In the next chapter I will show you how to set up your diet.

Chapter 6

A Typical Setup To Maximize Your Results

Okay, to the basics... To lose weight you have to eat less than you usually do. That's it. But what is less? You'll need to find your baseline maintenance amount of food - the amount of food you eat that maintains your current weight. Some people call this your "BMR" (basal metabolic rate); it's the amount of calories your body uses if you were to just lie in bed all day. Since you aren't lying in bed all day, you add a some extra calories to this to account for your usual daily activity.

There are mathematical formulas you can use to get a rough number, and they aren't 100% accurate, but that doesn't matter. All that matters is that you eat RELATIVELY less than you usually do. Now, I'm not going to ask you to do math, so go ahead and use Google and search "BMR Calculator" and pick one. Punch in the numbers and get your BMR.

My BMR is roughly 1900 calories. If I eat around that number, I'll stay the same weight.

To lose weight, you have to eat less than that. How much less? That's up to you, but I recommend not going any lower than ten times your goal weight. If your goal weight is 135, set your calories at no less than 1350. Eating 10 times your goal weight will have you losing 1-2 pounds per week. If you eat less than that you'll be causing yourself unnecessary stress and you'll eventually have a binge. You don't want that. You want this to be the last time you are dieting.

Okay, so now you have your "caloric deficit". That is the difference between your BMR and your diet limit.

What should you eat? Well, you should eat whatever you like to eat, within reason, but I recommend favoring protein and veggies, this will help keep you nice and satisfied. That's what's great about this way of eating, if you are vegetarian, continue being vegetarian, vegan, paleo, whatever you want, it's all about that caloric deficit.

How do you know you're eating at your deficit? I recommend using a calorie tracking tool for a few weeks so you know what you're consuming. The best app I have found is MyFitnessPal. Set up a free account and track everything you put in your mouth for 2 to 3 weeks. Try to eat a lot of the same meals, and eventually you'll be able to estimate calories by comparing it to your usual foods. For me, I don't have to track at all if I don't want to. My usual 1 large meal and 1 small meal keep me at my deficit and the weight falls off.

The last thing you need to remember has to do with weight loss stalls. You might find that your weight loss stops its usual rate. If it ever stops for more than 2 weeks, you've hit a plateau.

Don't panic!

This simply means your body has gotten used to the deficit and your hormones have signaled your body to hang on to the weight. All you need to do is take a 2 week "diet break" by eating at maintenance calories (remember the BMR from above?) Usually this just means eating a slightly larger second meal, for me anyway. After that, drop your calories again and you'll more than likely continue shedding weight.

Chapter 7

Concerns As A Woman

This chapter is short and sweet. And that's good news. You may have read elsewhere that only men get to reap the rewards of intermittent fasting. That for some reason, because women get pregnant, intermittent fasting causes all hell to break lose!

Now, do you really think eating later in the day would cause such a disaster?

Fortunately, that couldn't be further from the truth. I've found countless cases of women having identical benefits and results from intermittent fasting as men.

The only thing I have to say about this is that you should listen to your body and adapt this way of eating so that it works for YOU. After you have made that first 2 week adjustment (that period of time where you WILL be hungry because your hormones are adapted to eating in the morning) you should listen to your body and adapt. Pay attention to your work, are you getting spacey or grouchy with your co-workers? That's a good sign you should eat something. If that means you can't stretch your first meal out beyond 2pm, so be it. Eat!

Is your caloric deficit too small? Increase it! This is the best advice when it comes to dieting success. You don't want to be suffering and, for women, compared to men, this can mean choosing a wider window to eat in. Instead of a 16-hour fast, shorten it to 12-14 hours.

If a huge first meal makes you sleepy, eat 2 medium sized meals instead, or don't eat carbs until closer to bedtime.

One of the hidden benefits about intermittent fasting is increased intuition about what your body needs. Eating the old way, you barely have time to register that you are actually hungry. Intermittent fasting has attuned me to my true hunger signals, to when I'm truly satisfied and don't need any more.

Chapter 8

Exercise For Fun, Not As A Requirement

I've saved exercise for the latter half of the book because your diet is the NUMBER 1 thing you need to focus on to lose weight. It's where your effort should be directed most. The reason for this is simply a matter of practicality. You could go for a 1 hour brisk walk or simply NOT EAT that 400 calorie bagel and cream cheese.

Exercise is important for our health, that goes without saying, but for fat loss, it's secondary.

But for me, I have found that walking helps me to unwind, clear my head, and suppresses my appetite. For that reason, I think walking is the best thing you can do to help with your weight loss efforts. I like to walk for 40-60 minutes around lunchtime while everyone is sitting on their ass eating.

Another benefit is that, if you walk while fasting, your body will be converting your stored body fat into the energy source for your walk. Goodbye, body fat!

Remember, it isn't necessary for your fat loss efforts, so do it if you like to, or to give yourself some extra calories for some plans you have later. Want to have that gin and tonic tonight but don't have the calories left for your deficit? Go for a 40-minute brisk walk!

8.1 Strength Training

This last point I won't go too deep into, but it's important.

When you are on a fat loss diet, you will INEVITABLY lose muscle. Your body will be using a combination of fat and muscle protein for energy. You want to try to prevent your body from doing this. You don't want to be a muscle-less skeleton.

The best way to prevent this is to do some form of strength training. I'll let you decide what that is, but for me, I like to keep it as simple as possible and I think you should too. This means simple bodyweight calisthenics. No gym. Just push-ups, pull-ups, squats, dips, etc. I recommend you check out the book *Convict Conditioning* by Paul Wade for a crash course on the slow process of increasing your strength using only bodyweight training. Your body is all you need.

Chapter 9

Strategies That Make It Effortless

Alright, so you want to start doing this fasting thing but you have some concerns. "Won't I be starving and irritable?" "I don't want to go to jail for workplace violence..." Fortunately for you, after a week or so, the hunger pangs you usually have in the morning will shift to lunchtime (or later). But to make it easier, here are a some strategies you can use to make you an IF master.

9.1 Black Coffee

If you're like me, you drink coffee every morning, so this one will be easy for you. If you can, drink it black, this will keep your body in a fasted state. If you put milk or cream in it, your body will start to use that for energy instead of your body fat. Which would you rather occur?

The other benefit of coffee, and the one more relevant to this chapter, is that it blunts hunger. Try it, if you feel hungry, drink a cup or two of black coffee and see how you feel. I find it elevates my focus so I become a machine at work. No, not a robot, but a highly effective, clear-minded beast!

There are some hidden benefits related to caffeine increasing the amount of fat you burn while you're fasted, but you can find those with a simple google search. We aren't here to waste your time with citations. But, as usual, I like to stick with the more practical and obvious benefits, and those are hunger blunting and increasing productivity. Try it; you'll love it.

9.2 Seltzer Water

This one is similar to coffee— if you start to feel a little hungry, a little empty in the belly, try drinking a can of sparkling water. The zero calorie kind that is flavored is my favorite. I drink this cran-raspberry version from La Croix. The carbonation seems to take up space in your belly and kills the hunger.

I also just like to have a nice fizzy drink from time to time. Fresh water is great, but sometimes while I'm working, it's refreshing to sip a flavored beverage.

9.3 A Piece Of Fruit

Okay, so let's say you have made it all the way to lunch time fasted but you'd like to push it a little further. Sometimes I like to push my first meal a little further into the afternoon, like 3-5pm, but at this point, you're going to start feeling hungry, and, really, it's time to eat. For me though, I'm sometimes so focused on work that I'd rather not cook. Now is the time to grab a piece of fruit from the fridge. Maybe an apple or a peach.

Now, as I mentioned in regards to putting milk in your coffee, this is going to shift your body out of fasting mode, but that's okay, the point of eating now is, again, to blunt your hunger so that you have even more calories. Maybe it's a holiday and you're planning to really let loose at the dinner table. Use these strategies so that you have a large enough calorie buffer that you can eat all you want and still lose weight!

Remember though, you aren't trying to starve yourself, and if at any point you start to feel irritable, or start to notice a decline in your work, just eat. Listen to your body. For me, if I sometimes want to push my first meal until after work, I might start feeling a bit anxious towards the end of the day, so the fruit brings me back on point.

9.4 Meal Sizing

This last strategy is how you choose to split the size of your meals and is more of a personal preference. You must choose what works best for you.

9.4.1 One Large Meal And One Smaller Meal

The one large and one small meal strategy is what I've been using recently, because it allows me to have a massive meal for my first meal, which honestly keeps me satisfied to the point where I usually don't feel much hunger for the rest of the day.

I like it because it has simplified my life so much. I only have to prepare one meal per day, and then my second meal is practically a snack. A couple small quesadillas or a few eggs and a piece of toast. And if you wanted to you could swap your meals so the first one is small and then your dinnertime meal is the big one. Perfect for saving up your calories for a dinner date.

9.4.2 Two Medium-Sized Meals

I followed this strategy for a very long time and its greatest benefit is maintenance. If you like the weight you are at and just want to maintain it, have 2 medium-sized meals. What's a medium-sized meal? It's basically the usual amount of food you would eat for lunch or dinner, a standard plate of food.

You can even follow this plan to lose weight too, since you'll be cutting out breakfast and eating less. I tended not to lose weight because, as I mentioned earlier, I like food ... like a little too much. So my medium was a big medium...

9.4.3 Three Smaller Meals

Everyone is different, and some people are grazers. You like to munch on things here and there. A small salad here, maybe a granola bar, some fancy vegan cookies. Now, I'm not advocating cookies, but I know people that just don't eat big meals. It's too much for them. If they ate like I did they would be on the floor in pain.

The Three-Small-Meals plan is perfect for them. You've shifted your calories to the afternoon, and by grazing as usual, you'll have once again achieved that calorie deficit (eating less) you need to lose weight.

The problem with this style is that you might overgraze. At some point you need to know exactly how much food you put in your body on a typical day. Grazers tend to eat things that are more carb-centric or sugary, which your body uses up fast, leaving you hungry again quickly. That's why I suggest trying to eat a larger meal that has a good amount of fat to keep you nice and full.

If it works for you though then do it. Keep an eye on your weight and, if you see progress, you're good to go!

47884056R00015

Made in the USA
Middletown, DE
04 September 2017